I0427954

HEALTH STRATEGY: ESSENTIAL OILS FOR ESTHETICS

The content on these pages are owned, authored, and under intellectual copyright by Victoria Edge. No part of this Booklet may be duplicated or incorporated into any other work without express written permission. No exceptions will be permitted, and violators will be prosecuted to the fullest extent of the law

Health Strategy – Essential oils for Aesthetics

Copyright 2010 Victoria Edge

Reprint 2015 (revision 2)

The information offered in this book is for educational purposes and is not meant to substitute or replace the advice of a physician or other medical professional.
Please seek medical advice for any serious condition.

HEALTH STRATEGY: ESSENTIAL OILS FOR ESTHETICS

Victoria Edge

Contents

Introduction

My name is Victoria Edge. I have been working with essential oils for about 20 years now. I have conducted international workshops on using, blending and healing with essential oils. I work locally with herb shops, natural health providers, massage therapists and other holistic practitioners teaching, lecturing and consulting to bring more vibrant health to their customers and clients. My popular book, **Health Strategy: Essential Oils** has been a huge success for introducing the healing powers of essential oils to beginners and practitioners alike.

A few years back I began working with some local natural cosmetic spas, cosmetology schools and other esthetic leaders to develop recipes, processes and delivery methods for using the healing powers and constituent of essential oils to address signs of aging, dry skin, brittle hair, and other esthetic issues. The core material in this book comes from those reports, study guides, recipes, and guideline I developed for the esthetics industry.

Now those recipes, ideas and essential oil blends are available to you, in this information packed book, **Health Strategy: Essential oils for Esthetics**.

Acknowledgements:

I do want to thank my very dear friend, Erin Post ND, who has held my hand through my journey, guided, prodded and helped me test out many recipes! And thank you to my friend and beauty guru, Ginger Fortune, whose energy, strength and dedication to natural beauty, drove her to create her own natural line of cosmetics, Ginger Cosmetics, and whose inspiration, is woven throughout this book. Without these two amazing women, I would not be writing this book.

I also want to say thank you to my two kids, Alex and Katie. They have survived my trial and error and my failures. Our kitchen and my office often looked like a laboratory, and they often joked about my "potions" but they always knew that they would work.

Getting Started

Using essential oils for health and beauty can be traced back for centuries. The Egyptians used essential oils in incenses and as offerings to the gods. Cleopatra was well versed in the uses of essential oils for beauty and in cosmetics. Mental illnesses such as mania and depression were treated with these valuable oils, and of course they were used to adorn, cleanse and anoint the dead in their elaborate preservations process. Even today the excavated remains of the pharaohs' are still smell good!

The use of essential oils is well documented by the Greeks, who based many of their practices and techniques on those of the Egyptians. Hippocrates, known to most as the father of modern medicine, recommended regular aromatic baths and scented massage in order maintain health. The use of essential oils in the healing of wounds was practiced by another Greek physician, Megallus, and Dioscorides wrote of using medicinal plants in the ancient reference, De Materia Medica.

With so many chemicals in our world, in our food and in our cosmetics, we are all looking older than we need to. Making the switch to using high quality, pure and natural products in cosmetics, and beauty regimes can go a long way to stop and in some cases reverse the aging process.

One Word of Warning

Some people (less than 1%) have an allergy to some oils, so before you try any oil, apply it, mixed in water (1 drop oil to 1 Tbsp carrier oil), in a very small patch to the back of the hand and check it after a day or so. If it is red, or itches, do not continue use. Remember, essential oils are very concentrated and are far more potent than over the counter products. Also, keep in mind, unless specifically suggested, do not apply essential oils undiluted to skin (some oils are fine, but others are very strong), so best to be over cautious as you begin.

For Your Convenience

Blending, oil chemistry and common measurements also appear in my other book, ***Health Strategy: Essential Oils***, which I am reproducing here, for your convenience. Anytime you blend or begin working with oils, it is important to have some basic knowledge.

Blending

The following essential oil recipes can be modified to your own tastes (or sense of smell). Keep in mind the following tips when working with essential oils, and then, have fun and make up your own!

Essential Oil Blending Tips

Throughout this book, you will find recipes, oil combinations and other ideas for blending essential oils. When you are ready, feel free to come up with your own blends. Keep in mind the mixture may be therapeutic, but if the scent is not pleasant, it will not be easy to use. Keep these blending tips, equivalent measurements and general rules in mind if you plan to improvise.

In general:

- 2 – 8 drops of essential oil to 1 TBSP (1/2 oz) of Carrier
- A full body massage takes 1-2 ounces (6-12 teaspoons) of carrier oil
- **NEVER** use mineral oil or petroleum oil with essential oils (it destroys the properties)
- NEVER microwave oils to heat.
- **Never put oils in plastic cups or Styrofoam cups** as the oil will mark the plastic and dissolve the Styrofoam.

- In a pinch you can use Olive oil to blend essential oils. It is a bit heavier, but in some applications that works better than thinner.

Common Equivalent Measures

For your convenience, as you begin experimenting, you may want to substitute ingredients, multiply or divide the recipe for larger or smaller volume, you will need to know what equals what. So we have included the table below.

Common measures	Is equal to (Equivalent measures
1 ounce	2 tablespoons
	6 teaspoons
	30 milliliters (ml)
	900 drops of oil
1/2 ounce	1 tablespoon
	3 teaspoons
	15 milliliters (ml)
	450 drops of oil
1/3 ounce	2 teaspoons
	10 milliliters (ml)
	300 drops of oil
1/6 ounce	1 teaspoon
	5 milliliters (ml)
	100 drops of oil

A Quick Chemistry Lesson

You may not need to know this chemistry lesson, however, the table below helps to illustrate that these oils have medicinal chemical properties and from this list, you can learn to alternate or substitute one oil for another with a similar property.

Essential Plant Extract Oils can be classified into 7 chemical properties:

Oil Property Type	Chemical Properties
Alcohols	**Benefits**: antiseptic, antiviral properties and a slight uplifting quality. **Types**: *Linalol* (abundant in lavender), *citronellol* (found in rose, lemon, eucalyptus and geranium) and *geraniol* (geranium and palmarosa).
Aldehydes	**Benefits**: generally sedative, though uplifting, quality. Aldehydes are present in lemon-scented essences, such as citronella and lemongrass.
Esters	**Benefits**: fungicidal and sedative, usually with a fruity odor **Types**: *linalyl acetate* (clary sage and lavender), and *geranyl acetate* (sweet marjoram).
Ketones	**Benefits**: eases congestion and aid the flow of mucus, which is why plants and essences containing relatively large quantities of these substances are usually helpful for upper respiratory complaints. **Types**: thujone, pulegone, jasmone, fenchone **Cautions**: Some ketones (such as thujone), are known to be toxic, Oils containing such ketones should be used with caution by most lay people, such as Mugwort, tansy, wormwood and common sage contain the potentially risky thujone. Non-toxic ketones include jasmone, found in jasmine, and fenchone in sweet fennel.
Oxides	**Benefits**: expectorant effect Types: camphoraceous such as rosemary, eucalyptus, meleleuca and cajuput.

Phenols	**Benefits**: bactericidal with a strong, stimulating effect on the central nervous system. **Types**: eugenol, thymol, carvacrol, anethole, estragole **Cautions**: Oils containing relatively large quantities of eugenol, thymol or carvacrol are potentially irritating to skin and mucous membranes, such as clove, thyme and oregano. Oils with anethole (from fennel) and estragole (tarragon) are not at all caustic.
Terpenes	**Benefits**: remarkable anti-inflammatory and bactericidal properties **Types**: limonene pinene chamazulene farnesol. Due to the wide variety of properties, it is difficult to make overly simplified statements about their therapeutic actions. However, common terpenes include limonene (an antiviral agent found in 90 per cent of citrus oils), and pinene (an antiseptic found in high concentrations in pine and turpentine oils). Others, such as chamazulene and farnesol (found in chamomile essence),

General Oils To Use For Specific Purposes

You can use the recipes in this book and modify them using specific oils for specific purposes. For example, you can use the Eye Cream recipe and add or substitute a oil or blend of oils found under the Wrinkles category to focus the purpose or your cream.

If you thought essential oils were beneficial only for those suffering from certain ailments or body pains, think again. Another reason why it has been widely popular from various parts of the world is because of its ability to provide cosmetic benefits. Since the days of Cleopatra, young and older people alike have experienced its excellent ability to preserve natural beauty, if not enhance it.

Essential Oils for Facial Care

Facial care is one of the first areas in cosmetics that every individual, men and women, look into. Indeed, their face is the most noticeable feature and it only makes sense that you take proper care of it. There are a whole variety of essential oil types that can preserve and enhance the natural beauty of your face.

Essential Oils for use with Specific Skin Conditions			
For normal skin:	For dry skin:	For oily skin:	For wrinkles
Geranium	Lavender	Cypress	Frankincense
Frankincense	Patchouli	Frankincense	Myrrh
Lavender	Sandalwood	Clary sage	Rose
Jasmine	Rosemary	Lavender	Lavender
Rose	Rose	Lemon	Patchouli
Lemon		Myrrh	Sandalwood
Wild orange		Thyme	Clary sage
		Wild orange	
		Rosemary	
		Lime	

Essential Oils for Hair Care

Your hair is considered as your crowning glory. It is also a reflection of your own health status; hence, a healthy hair indicates a healthy you. On the next page are some types of hair and the recommended essential oils for use in treating and caring for your specific hair type:

Essential Oils for use with Specific Hair Conditions				
Normal hair:	Dry hair:	Oily hair:	Hair loss:	For Dandruff:
Lavender	Rosemary	Lemon	Ylang ylang	Basil
Geranium	Sandalwood	Lemongrass	Basil	Cypress
Eucalyptus	Geranium	Clary sage	Cypress	Lemon
Rosemary	Lavender	Cypress	Lemon	Meleleuca
Lemon		Basil	Clary sage	Rosemary
			Rosemary	Thyme
			Thyme	
			Peppermint	

Hair Care Recipes with Essential Oils

It's important to apply essential oils to your hair. Due to the effects of chemicals used in hair care products and hair dyes, many people suffer from a sensitive scalp.

Using essential oils can help calm the skin down and make hair look healthy again. Your hair will benefit from a treatment with any of these oils even if there are no significant hair or scalp issues to cure.

The best essential oils for hair can be used as often as needed, unlike many chemical hair treatment products. These essential oils suitable for several hair problems, such as: Dry skin on the scalp, Split hair ends , Dry and dull hair , Very thin or fine hair.

Carrier Oils for Hair

Always remember that you can use these essential oils (Pure, High quality oils) for hair direct to your hair, but to cover more surface, you can mix with carrier oils first.

Carrier oils that have a benefit to hair	
Carrier Oil	Benefit
Olive Oil	This oil can be combined with other nice smelling essential oils. Olive oil is especially beneficial for dry hair suffering from indoor heating and sun. The hair is nourished and will regain its elasticity after a treatment with this oil. Apply the oil to towel dry hair and leave on for at least half an hour.
Jojoba Oil	Jojoba oil can be used with any hair and skin type. Extremely damaged or breaking hair will benefit from the healing qualities of jojoba oil. This truly is one of the best essential oils for hair loss due to breakage. The oil can be applied as described before and a very small amount applied to the skin of the face will help prevent hair dye stains when dye is applied.
Carrot Oil	Carrot oil is also marketed as a cosmetic due to its excellent regenerative, cleansing and detoxifying properties and has been shown to improve the appearance and texture of skin and hair, no doubt in large part to its high vitamin content, The antioxidants in carrot oil also protect against damage caused by excessive exposure to UV radiation from the sun, which is why carrot oil is used as an active ingredient in many sun protection products.

Recipes for Hair

Hair conditioner
1 tbsp Jojoba carrier oil
3 drops Rosemary

Mix the Jojoba and Rosemary in a small bowl (tiny condiment bowls work great for this). Wet your hair with warm water and then apply the conditioner. Let it sit on your hair for 15-30 minutes. Then, wash your hair as normal. Jojoba and rosemary are helpful for dry hair. The rosemary is also said to be helpful in aiding dandruff.

Scented Hair
2 drops of Rosemary or Lavender oils

Apply to the bristles of your hairbrush and brush your hair well. The oils will leave your hair with a wonderful aroma.

De–Tangle Conditioning Hair Spray
4 oz distilled water
20 drops Virgin carrot oil
20 drops Lavender
20 drops Rosemary
1 tsp aloe vera (as emulsifier)

Put distilled water in a spray bottle. Add emulsifier and shake well, then add oils and shake again thoroughly. Use when hair is wet or dry. Spray enough to slightly dampen hair (if it is dry) and gently brush or comb hair. De tangles and conditions hair without leaving any residue. For some hair it may also control frizziness

Hair Loss Recipe
1 tbsp Jojoba
1 tbsp Sweet almond
1 tsp Virgin carrot oil
10 drops Lavender oil
6 drops Clary Sage
4 drops Roman Chamomile
4 drops Rosemary
Blend all ingredients in a clean bottle. Shake well and warm before using. Apply a few drops into scalp, leave overnight or until absorbed in. Apply several times a week.

Bath Recipes Using Essential Oils

Taking a bath can be all things to all people. Depending on your choice of herbs, a bath or shower can help you face the rigors of the day or relax afterwards. Not only that, a bath can help soften the skin and replenish the body's natural oils.

Frothy Bath Oil

2 eggs
1 cup olive oil
1/2 cup corn oil
1/2 cup almond oil
1 cup milk
2 Tbsp clear honey
1 cup milk
1/2 cup vodka
1 Tbsp mild soap flakes
3 drops essential oil of your choice

Beat together the eggs, vegetable oils, and honey. Add the milk, vodka, soap flakes, and essential oil, still beating. Pour into bottles, cover, label and store in the refrigerator.

Add about one tbsp under the faucet when running the water for a warm bath.

Floral Bath Gel

3 Tbsp fresh or dried flowers, picked from the stalks
1/2 cup spring water
12 Tbsp grated castile soap
3-4 drops essential oil of choice

Pound the flowers with a mortar and pestle until they form a paste or powder. Put the water into a small pan and bring to a boil. Beat in the grated soap until it has dissolved, then remove pan from heat. Stir in the flowers and essential oil.

Leave to cool, then pour into bottles, cover, label and store in the refrigerator. Use as a soft soap.

Bath Salts

Bath salts, due to their mineral content, relax mind body and soul, soothe sore muscles and soothe the skin.

Simple Lavender Bath Salts

1 1/2 cups Dead Sea Salts
4-6 drops of lavender essential oil

Combine salts and essential oil, and stir well. Put in pint canning jar and label. Let set for 12 hours.

Muscle Relaxing Bath Salts

4 cups Epsom Salts
40 drops total of Roman Chamomile, lavender, clary sage, basil, Marjoram and/or Rosemary essential oils

Makes 4 uses. Combine salts and essential oil, and blend well. Put in mason jar and label. Let set for 12 hours. Use One cup per bath

Skin Care Recipes Using Essential Oils

Making your own skin Recipes is itself a pleasurable pastime. Just to stir a handful of pot marigold petals into a bowl of steaming water is both invigorating and calming, an indirect form of Aromatherapy. The following recipes offers therapeutic and cosmetic blends to help you care for your skin or just to allow a little self indulgence.

Purifying Masks

This is a purifying, toning, soothing, and rejuvenating mask. The basic ingredients are:
Basic Mask Mix:
2 ounces Green Clay
3 tsp Cornflour

Mix together and keep in a jar, ready for combining in one of the formulas below.

Purifying Mask - Normal Skin

1 Tbsp Basic Mask Mix
1 Egg Yolk
1 tsp water
1 drop Geranium essential oil
1 drop Rose

Blend the ingredients together to form a smooth paste. Apply in a thin layer to face, avoiding eye area. Leave on the skin for fifteen minutes. Rinse off and apply a moisturizer or facial oil. Dab the face with a tissue.

Purifying Mask - Dry Skin

1 Tbsp Basic Mask Mix
1 Egg Yolk
1 tsp Almond or Evening Primrose Oil
1/4 tsp Virgin carrot Oil
2 tsp water
1 drop Chamomile essential oil
1 drop Rose essential oil

Blend the ingredients together to form a smooth paste. Apply in a thin layer to face, avoiding eye area. Leave on the skin for fifteen minutes. Rinse off and apply a moisturizer or facial oil. Dab the face with a tissue.

Purifying Mask - Oily Skin

1 Tbsp Basic Mask Mix
1 Tbsp Brewer's Yeast
1 Tbsp Water
1 drop of Rosemary essential oil
1 drop of Lavender essential oil

Blend the ingredients together to form a smooth paste. Apply in a thin layer to face, avoiding eye area. Leave on the skin for fifteen minutes. Rinse off and apply a moisturizer or facial oil. Dab the face with a tissue.

Revitalizing Mask for Dehydrated Skin

1 Tbsp Basic Mask Mix
1 Egg Yolk
1 tsp Brewer's Yeast
1 tsp Jojoba Oil
1/4 tsp virgin carrot oil
1 Tbsp Water
1 drop Chamomile essential oil

Blend the ingredients together to form a smooth paste. Apply in a thin layer to face, avoiding eye area. Leave on the skin for fifteen minutes. Rinse off and apply a moisturizer or facial oil. Dab the face with a tissue.

Mask for Acne

1 tbsp Basic Mask Mix
1 tsp Water
1 drop of Chamomile essential oil
1 drop of Lavender essential oil
1 drop Eucalyptus essential oil and
1 drop Patchouli essential oil

Blend the ingredients together to form a smooth paste. Apply in a thin layer to face, avoiding eye area. Leave on the skin for fifteen minutes. Rinse off and apply a moisturizer or facial oil. Dab the face with a tissue.

Cosmetic Face Lotions, Serums, and Creams

Facial Scrub (not for sensitive skin)

1 tbsp ground oatmeal
1 tbsp ground dried lavender blossoms
1 tbsp ground thyme leaves
1 tbsp ground almonds
4 drops lemon essential oil

Grind all dry ingredients finely and mix until uniform. Add essential oil and mix well. Store in a glass container. Use 1 1/2 tsp with enough water to make a paste. Gently massage into skin and rinse thoroughly.

Nourishing Facial Serum

1/2 ounce jojoba oil
1/4 ounce evening primrose oil
1/4 tsp virgin carrot oil
15 drops vitamin E oil
8 drops geranium essential oil
8 drops frankincense essential oil

Combine oils in a 1 ounce dark glass bottle that has a lid with a dropper, cap the bottle, and invert it several times to mix. Only 1 or 2 drops of serum should be used for the entire face and throat area, either on its own or before applying facial lotion.

Night Cream

3 tbsp olive oil
1 tbsp aloe vera gel
1 tbsp shea butter
2 tsp grated beeswax
1 tbsp rosewater
1/4 tsp lecithin
oil from two capsules of vitamin E
3 drops chamomile or lavender essential oil

Combine olive oil, and vitamin E, butter, and beeswax in a quart size glass mason jar with a lid and place this in a small saucepan of water until melted. Bring water to a boil, stirring ingredients constantly until smooth.

Remove from heat just before beeswax is completely melted. Finish melting by stirring in warm oil. Add the vitamin E oil and lecithin and stir in between additions. Mix rosewater and aloe together and slowly add to main mixture. Continue stirring with a small metal whisk. Once mixture is cooled, add the essential oil and stir. Store inside drawer or cabinet. Try to keep away from sun and heat. Use nightly-especially in cold or dry weather.

Scented Toner

5 drops lavender essential oil (alternate – lemon or wild orange essential oil)
5 drops peppermint essential oil
8 oz witch hazel

Add essential oils to witch hazel. Pour into sterilized bottle. Apply with cotton ball morning and evening after cleansing and before moisturizing.

Lotion Bars

1 oz beeswax
1 oz cocoa butter
1 oz olive oil
20 drops total of essential oil (Suggested oils: lavender, chamomile, wild orange, rosemary, sandalwood, vetiver, white fir, bergamot, Ylang Ylang)
(to increase proportions, use equal parts wax, butter and olive oil and 20 drops of Essential oil per 3 oz of oils)

Combine beeswax in a quart size glass mason jar with a lid and place this in a small saucepan of water until melted. Bring water to a boil, stirring ingredients constantly until smooth.

Add cocoa butter and olive oil. Stir until butter is entirely melted and oils are mixed. Allow to cool slightly, add essential oils. Pour into molds and allow to harden.

Moisturizing Jelly

2 ounces olive oil
1/2 ounce grated beeswax
12 drops grapefruit seed extract

Combine the olive oil and beeswax, in a quart size glass mason jar with a lid and place this in a small saucepan of water until melted. Bring water to a boil, stirring ingredients constantly until smooth.

Remove mixture from the heat and add the grapefruit seed extract. Beat with a hand mixer until creamy. Makes 1/4 cup. Store in a glass jar with a screw-top. This jelly will keep for a year.

Massage Butter

2 tbsp. coconut oil
2 tbsp. cocoa butter
2 tbsp. apricot kernel oil
1 1/4 tsp. beeswax
20 drops total Essential oil (Suggested oils: lavender, chamomile, wild orange, rosemary, sandalwood, vetiver, white fir, bergamot, Ylang Ylang)

Melt all the ingredients together over low heat. Remove from heat and cool slightly. Add essential oil, stir thoroughly. Pour into containers and label.

Face Cream

1/2 tsp. (.10 ounce) beeswax
1 1/2 tsp. coconut oil
1 3/4 tsp. cocoa butter
1/4 tsp. lanolin
2 tbsp. distilled water
3 tbsp. almond oil
1 3/4 tsp. rose water
3/4 tsp. glycerin
1 tbsp. aloe vera gel
1 drop meleleuca essential oil
3 drops lavender essential oil
3 drops frankincense essential oil

Melt the oils, cocoa butter, beeswax and lanolin slowly in double boiler. Remove from heat and allow mixture to cool to room temperature. Add room temperature distilled water, rose water, glycerin, aloe vera and essential oils into a blender. Blend medium high and slowly add room temperature oil mixture. The mixture should look thick and creamy. Pour 2 week's worth of cream mixture into containers and label. Store extra containers in refrigerator.

Mature Skin - Orange Blossom Cleansing Cream

2 tbsp jojoba oil
1 tbsp almond oil
1tbsp coconut oil
1 tbsp grated beeswax
1 400IU Vitamin E capsule (optional)
80mls rosewater
3 drops sandalwood essential oil
3 drops wild orange essential oil
3 drops grapefruit seed extract (optional - preservative)

In a quart size glass mason jar with a lid warm the oils and add the beeswax. Gently heat the oils and wax until the wax is dissolved-do not overheat. Add the vitamin E capsule (acts as a preservative) contents, and then stir in the rosewater slowly-trickle it in. Keep stirring the cream until you are sure it has all emulsified and then add the essential oils and grapefruit seed extract (which acts as a preservative and will give the product a shelf life of up to two years). Bring water to a low boil, stirring ingredients constantly until smooth. Remove from heat and pour into desired pots or tins.

Revitalizing Cream

3 tbsp almond oil
1 tbsp coconut oil
1 tbsp grated beeswax
1 400IU capsule Vit-E (optional)
60mls rosewater
3 drops wild orange oil
3 drops sandalwood oil
3 drops grapefruit seed extract (optional - preservative)

In a quart size glass mason jar with a lid warm the oils and add the beeswax. Gently heat the oils and wax until the wax is dissolved-do not overheat. Add the vitamin E capsule (acts as a preservative) contents, and then stir in the rosewater slowly-trickle it in. Keep stirring the cream until you are sure it has all emulsified and then add the essential oils and grapefruit seed extract (which acts as a preservative and will give the product a shelf life of up to two years). Bring water to a low boil, stirring ingredients constantly until smooth. Remove from heat and pour into desired pots or tins.

Soothing Astringent

250mls witch hazel
10 drops eucalyptus oil
10 drops lavender oil

Mix ingredients together in a glass bottle and shake well.

Eye Cream

1 tbsp lanolin
2 tsp almond oil
2 tsp wheatgerm oil
1 tsp apricot oil
2 tsp purified water
5 drops lavender essential oil
3 drops frankincense essential oil

Melt the oils and lanolin in a double boiler until the mixture is liquid but not overheated. Warm the water in a separate container to the same temp as the oil mixture and slowly trickle the water into the oils. Stir constantly until cool and spoon into sterilized jars and cap immediately.

Anti Aging Eye Serum Recipe Restorative

1 ounce jojoba oil
5 drops sandalwood essential oil
3 drops frankincense oil
5 drops rose essential oil

Combine essential oils with Jojoba oil and store in a one-ounce glass bottle with a dropper top.

Apply 1 drop of the oil to your finger and gently smooth the oil beneath your eye and onto the area just beneath the brow bone. Do not apply oil directly to your eyelids.

Jojoba Eye Wrinkle Cream

3 tsp. jojoba oil
3 tsp. apricot-kernel oil
1 tsp. beeswax
5 tsp. rose water
1/4 tsp. borax
5 drops virgin carrot oil
3 drops rose or myrrh essential oil
3 drops frankincense

Combine jojoba oil, apricot-kernel oil and beeswax in a quart size glass mason jar with a lid and place this in a small saucepan of water until melted.   Bring water to a boil, stirring ingredients constantly until smooth.

Remove from heat and stir to blend. While that is cooling, in another small mason jar, warm the rose water over very low heat and add the borax; stir until the borax is dissolved, and remove from heat. Borax acts as a natural preservative. Allow to cool to medium luke warm temp. Add to borax/rose water in the oil wax blend. Rapidly stir wax and virgin carrot oil and rose water and borax mixture. Allow to cool to room temp then add the essential oils.

Put the finished eye cream into a clean glass cosmetic jar.

Apply the cream under your eyes and leave for about 10 minutes; wipe off the excess cream with a soft cloth. Apply each morning and evening before moisturizing.

Ultimate Eye Serum
1 tbsp olive oil
1 tsp pomegranate seed oil
1/4 tsp virgin carrot oil
1 tsp cranberry seed oil
3 drops pachouli essential oil

Combine oils and store in a one-ounce glass bottle with a dropper top. Apply 1 drop of the oil to your finger and gently smooth the oil around eye area at night. Less is more!

Eye Wrinkle Cream
3 tsp. jojoba oil
3 tsp. apricot-kernel oil
1 tsp. cranberry seed oil
1/4 tsp. virgin carrot oil
1 tsp. beeswax
5 drops sandalwood essential oil
3 drops frankincense essential oil

Melt beeswax and oils. Stir, cool to room temp. Add virgin carrot oil. Pour into jar. Apply to your finger and gently smooth the oil around eye area at night. Less is more!

Aloe Vera Eye Cream
1 tsp apricot kernel oil
1 tsp grapefruit seed essential oil
1 tsp grated beeswax
1/2 tsp aloe vera gel
contents of 1 vitamin E capsule
5 drops rose oil

Combine oil and Beeswax in a quart size glass mason jar with a lid and place this in a small saucepan of water until melted. Bring water to a boil, stirring ingredients constantly until smooth.

Remove from the heat. Using a wooden spoon, mix in the aloe gel. Allow to cool to lukewarm temp and add essential oil and Vitamin E (puncture the capsule and squeeze out its contents), stir well. Pour into a small glass jar. Cool and cap tightly. Apply nightly before bed.

Lavender Eye Serum
3 Tbsp. Jojoba oil
1 Tbsp. olive oil
5 drops lavender essential oil
3 drops Roman chamomile essential oil
2 drops bergamot essential oil

Mix these oils in a glass eye dropper jar. Shake well before each use. Take one drop and gently apply to eye area before bedtime. This can also be used as an all over facial serum.

Anti Wrinkle Eye Serum Recipe for younger women
2 tbsp hazelnut oil
15 drops jojoba oil
3 drop lavender essential oil
3 drop pachouli essential oil
9 drops clary sage oil
2 capsules vitamin E

Mix these oils in a glass eye dropper jar. Shake well before each use. Take one drop and gently apply to eye area before bedtime.

Vitamin E Eye Serum Recipe
2 tbsp hazelnut oil
6 drops evening primrose oil
6 drops lavender essential oil
9 drops clary sage essential oil
contents of 1 vitamin E capsule

Mix these oils in a glass eye dropper jar. Shake well before each use. Take one drop and gently apply to eye area before bedtime.

Nail Care Recipes Using Essential Oils

Nail Massage Oil

4 ml pure jojoba and sweet almond oil base
2 drops each lemon, sandalwood, lavender, meleleuca,
contents of 1 vitamin E capsule punctured and squeezed into the
bottle

Combine all the ingredients and mix well. (unscented hand lotion
or cream may be substituted for the oil base.) Apply 2 drops of this
oil to each nail and 4 droops to each hand and massage in. The
massage is as important as the blend. It stimulates circulation and
relaxes hands that have been busy all day. This blend works equally
well on toenails.

Aromatic nail treatment

4 ounces liquid castile soap
30 drops total essential oils of lemon, lavender, eucalyptus or your
own blend

Combine soap and essential oils in a lotion or hand soap pump
bottle. Add a pump or two of soap to a moistened nail brush and
work up a good lather, then rinse thoroughly. Push the cuticle back
gently with a hand towel.

Hand Care Recipes Using Essential Oils

Foaming Hand Soap
1/3 cup Liquid unscented Castile soap
2/3 cup filtered water
20 drops total essential oil - lavender, clove, peppermint,
and/or lemon
A foaming soap dispenser

Pour the Castile soap and the essential oil into the jar and stir to combine. Fill the jar the rest of the way up with water. Screw on the lid and pump away!

Super Moisturizing Hand lotion
1/2 cup Almond or olive oil
1/4 cup coconut oil
1/4 beeswax
1 teaspoon Vitamin E oil
30 drops total of Essential Oils, lavender, rose, clove, or blend your own

Combine in a quart size glass mason jar with a lid and place this in a small saucepan of water until melted. Bring water to a boil, stirring ingredients constantly until smooth.

Remove from heat and add the essential oils.

Gently stir by hand until essential oils are incorporated.

Carefully pour into whatever jar or tin you will use for storage. This is a thicker moisturizing lotion, not suitable for pump jars.

Gentle, Natural, non-drying Hand Sanitizer

12 drops Lavender oil
6 drops Peppermint oil
3 ounces Aloe Vera gel
1 ounce Witch Hazel
1 capsule of Vitamin E (400 IUs)

First, mix together the oils and witch hazel. Then, add the aloe vera and blend thoroughly until all ingredients are well blended and the mixture is thick. Pour the mixture into a bottle. Shake vigorously before each use.

Foot Care Recipes Using Essential Oils

Foot Bath And Powder Recipes

Foot baths are especially helpful in treating tired, aching feet, cases of ingrown toe nails, foot fungus problems such as athlete's foot or ringworm, injuries or sprains.

Foot bath blends usually contain 8 to 10 drops of essential oils to 2 gallons of warm water. One cup of Epsom or sea salts can be added as well.

Aromatic Foot Powder

1/2 cup arrowroot (or an equal part blend of baking soda, cornstarch and clay)
8 drops essential oils of your choice (Suggested Oils: Any of the foot bath recipe blends or; cypress (especially useful for sweaty feet), pine, eucalyptus, ylang-ylang, grapefruit, patchouli, and frankincense are all suitable.)

Combine the arrowroot and essential oil, crushing the small clumps of oil between your fingers to evenly distribute them. This is made only with pure essential oils, no base oil is added. Be sure to wash you hands after handling pure essential oils to avoid any contact with the eyes or delicate mucous membranes.

Find an airtight container, preferably with a closable shaker top (like a baby powder bottle. Pry off the top, add the powder, then replace the top. Aromatic foot powder is nice sprinkled in socks, tennis shoes, and boots to keep the feet dry and cozy.

Tired Feet Bath
3 drops lavender
3 drops rosemary
4 drops lemon

Add oils to 2 gallons of warm water and mix well. This blend comes in handy when you've been on your feet all day. The lavender soothes the feet and the rosemary and lemon refresh, revive, and stimulate circulation.

Athlete's Foot Bath
4 drops meleleuca
4 drops lavender
2 drops sandalwood

Add oils to 1 gallon warm water and mix well. This combination of pure essential oils works wonders for people plagued with chronic athlete's foot problems. Meleleuca is anti-fungal, as is lavender. The sandalwood conditions, softens and soothes sore, cracked feet and toes. Its antiseptic and soothing properties help keep feet safe from secondary problems that can arise from the open cracked skin. Patchouli could be substituted for the sandalwood as a skin regenerator. Patchouli also has fungicidal properties.

Burning Foot Bath
3 drops peppermint
4 drops lavender
3 drops Roman chamomile

Add oils to 1 gallon of warm water and mix well. This blend is great for hot, weary feet that have been on the move all day. The peppermint cools and the lavender and chamomile soothe both feet and spirit.

Lotions, Gels and Bars

Lotions are emollients that can be absorbed into the skin to increase the moisture, decrease dryness and improve skin condition.

Deodorant Lotion

3 oz witch hazel
1 tsp glycerin
30 drops clary sage oil
10 drops lavender oil
10 drops thyme oil
10 drops patchouli oil
5 drops sandalwood oil

Blend all the ingredients together in a 125ml bottle. Shake well to mix and leave for four days before using. Shake before use.

Sunburn Relief Gel

2 Tbsp. Aloe Vera gel
5 drops lavender essential oil

Mix essential oil with aloe and put directly on sunburned or mildly irritated skin. If skin is too sensitive to touch, add enough water to make mixture sprayable (2 ounces) put in a spray bottle and spray on skin – let air dry.

Sunscreen Lotion Bar (approximately 15 spf)

1/2 cup shea butter
5 Tbsp beeswax
1/2 cup coconut oil
2 Tbsp non-nano Zinc Oxide powder
½ tsp Vitamin E Oil
30 drops total of Lavender essential oil and/or any non-citrus oil from chart on page 18

Combine in a quart size glass mason jar with a lid and place this in a small saucepan of water until melted. Bring water to a boil, stirring ingredients constantly until smooth.

Remove from heat and stir in the zinc oxide, the essential oil, and the vitamin E oil. Pour into small single use size silicone molds and place in the fridge to cool for about 30 minutes. Pop out and store in tins or an airtight container. Store at room temperature. Use caution as they will melt in the heat of the sun, but return to solid at room temperature.

Relaxing Aromatherapy Body Lotion

3 drops Lavender essential oil
2 drops Frankincense essential oil
4 drop Wild Orange essential oil
8 oz unscented body lotion

In an 8 ounce bottle add unscented body lotion, add the oils, cap the bottle, and shake it thoroughly.

Lotion bars

¼ cup coconut oil
¼ cup shea butter, cocoa butter or mango butter (or a mix of all three)
¼ cup beeswax
½ teaspoon Vitamin E oil
40 drops total of Lavender and Eucalyptus, peppermint and lemon, or your own blend.

Combine in a quart size glass mason jar with a lid and place this in a small saucepan of water until melted. Bring water to a boil, stirring ingredients constantly until smooth.

Remove from heat and add the essential oils.

Gently stir by hand until essential oils are incorporated.

Carefully pour into silicone molds. Allow the lotion bars to cool completely before attempting to pop out of molds.

Making Your Own Lip Balms

Advanced Cosmetic Recipe: Fresh Breath Lip Balm

2 tbsp Canola oil
1 tsp beeswax granules
10 drops vitamin E oil
3 drops Peppermint essential oil

Add beeswax in a quart size glass mason jar with a lid and place this in a small saucepan of water until melted. Bring water to a boil, stirring constantly until melted.

Stir the canola oil and vitamin E oil into the melted beeswax. Remove from the heat, quickly add the peppermint oil and stir. Before the mixture starts to cool and harden, pour it into empty lip balm containers. Allow the lip balm to harden and cool, then cap the lip balm containers.

Lip Repair

3 tsp grated beeswax
3 tsp avocado oil
1 tsp glycerin
1/8 tsp lecithin
1/2 tsp honey
contents of two vitamin E capsules
4 drops meleleuca essential oil
5 drops grapefruit essential oil

Combine beeswax in avocado oil in a quart size glass mason jar with a lid and place this in a small saucepan of water until melted. Bring water to a boil, stirring ingredients constantly until smooth.

Remove from heat and add vitamin E and lecithin. Combine honey and glycerin and then add to mixture. Finally, add essential oils. This will start setting right away so have a glass jar ready.

Simple Lip Balm

1 1/2 ounces cocoa butter
1 1/2 ounces grated beeswax
3 ounces olive oil
8 drops white fir, lime, lemon or wild orange essential oil

Melt the cocoa butter and beeswax slowly in a quart size glass mason jar with a lid and place this in a small saucepan of water until melted. Bring water to a boil, stirring ingredients constantly until smooth.

Add olive oil and stir well. Cool slightly add essential oil, then pour into containers.

For a softer balm, add more oil. For a harder balm, add more beeswax.

Honey Lip Saver Balm

1/2 tsp. beeswax
contents of 1 vitamin E capsule
2 tsp. olive oil
1/2 tsp. cocoa butter
1/2 tsp. honey
3 drops essential oil (suggested oils: Meleleuca for chapped lips or cold sores, lavender or wild orange for healing chapped lips)

Combine olive oil, beeswax and cocoa butter in a quart size glass mason jar with a lid and place this in a small saucepan of water until melted. Bring water to a boil, stirring ingredients constantly until smooth.

Remove from heat cool slightly. Stir in contents of the vitamin

Rose and Jojoba Lip Balm

This recipe will yield a soft and supple lip balm with plenty of glide. It's a balm that's good for everyday lip care or to apply under your lip color. The rose and jojoba oil are especially nourishing for older lips.
2 tsp beeswax
2 tbsp jojoba oil
8 drops Rose Absolute or Rose Otto Essential Oil

Combine beeswax and jojoba in a quart size glass mason jar with a lid and place this in a small saucepan of water until melted. Bring water to a boil, stirring ingredients constantly until smooth.

Remove bowl from simmering water and stir in rose oil. Stir and pour into an empty lip balm tube or small salve container. Cap and allow to set before applying.

Meleleuca Lip Balm with Orange-Mint Flavor

This recipe will yield a protective meleleuca sheen and powerfully fresh flavor punch.
2 tsp beeswax
2 tbsp jojoba oil
3 drops each of Peppermint and Wild Orange Essential Oils
2 drops Meleleuca Essential Oil

Measure beeswax and jojoba in a quart size glass mason jar with a lid and place this in a small saucepan of water until melted. Bring water to a boil, stirring ingredients constantly until smooth.

Remove bowl from simmering water and add essential oils. Stir and pour into an empty lip balm tube or small salve container. Cap and allow to set before applying.

Sugar and Salt Scrubs

Salts and Sugar scrubs are a luxurious way to pamper your skin since they exfoliate and moisturize at the same time and will leave your skin feeling smooth and soft. Most of the recipes listed here are for one treatment or use.

Lavender & Patchouli Scrub

1 cup brown sugar
1/4 cup almond oil
1/2 tsp vitamin E
6 drops patchouli essential oil
4 drops lavender essential oil

Latte Sugar Scrub with Coffee

1 tsp ground coffee
1 tsp sugar
2 drops cinnamon essential oil

Milk, Olive oil & Honey & Chamomile Sugar scrub

3 tbsp whole milk
2 cups white sugar
1/2 tsp extra virgin olive oil
1 tbsp dark organic honey
3 drops Roman chamomile essential oil

Aloe vera & Olive oil & Frankincense Sugar scrub

1/4 cup brown sugar
1 tbsp extra virgin olive oil
1 tbsp Aloe vera gel
3 drops Frankincense essential oil

Grapefruit, Aloe Vera, Jojoba & Olive Oil Sugar Scrub

1 cup white sugar
2 tbsp fresh grapefruit juice
2 drops grapefruit essential oil
4 tbsp Jojoba oil
2 tbsp extra virgin Olive oil
2 tbsp Aloe vera gel

Coconut Oil, Sea Salt, Lemon Juice & Honey Sugar Scrub

4 tbsp brown sugar
4 tbsp sea salt
1 tbsp coconut oil
1 tbsp fresh lemon juice
3 drops lime essential oil
2 drops lemon essential oil
1 tbsp dark organic Honey

Coffee & Brown Sugar Scrub

1/4 cup packed brown sugar
1/4 cup white sugar
3 tbsp fresh coffee grounds
5 tsp almond oil
4 drops roman chamomile essential oil

Coconut Oil, Sweet Orange, Lime & Vitamin E Oil Sugar Scrub

1/4 brown sugar
4 tbsp coconut oil
3 drops Sweet orange essential oil
2 drops lime essential oil
6 drops vitamin E oil
5 tsp jojoba oil
2 tsp honey
1 tsp vitamin E
1 tsp vanilla
2 drops peppermint essential oil

Honey & Orange juice Sugar scrub

1 tbsp dark organic Honey
4 tbsp Sugar (brown and/or white)
1/2 fresh orange (squeezed with pulp and juice)
2 drops wild orange essential oil
1 drop clove essential oil

Yogurt Sugar Scrub

3 tbsp Almond oil
1 tbsp yogurt
1 tbsp white sugar
3 drops Balance blend essential oil

Mix ingredients and use as a body scrub/exfoliation aid.

Wet your hands with warm water, dip the palms of your hands in sugar and gently rub in circular motions. Gently massage and exfoliate your skin. Wait 10 minutes, then wet hands and massage again taking the dead skin cells off. Rinse thoroughly.

Notes

Notes

www.ingramcontent.com/pod-product-compliance
Lightning Source LLC
Chambersburg PA
CBHW070816290526
45795CB00002B/734